T0252097

Thieme

Time and Life Management for Medical Students and Residents

Michael Sabel, MD
Professor
Department of Neurosurgery
University Hospital Düsseldorf
Düsseldorf, Germany

24 illustrations

Thieme
Stuttgart • New York • Delhi • Rio de Janeiro

Library of Congress Cataloging-in-Publication Data is available from the publisher.

© 2017 by Georg Thieme Verlag KG

Thieme Publishers Stuttgart
Rüdigerstrasse 14, 70469 Stuttgart, Germany
+49 [0]711 8931 421, customerservice@thieme.de

Thieme Publishers New York
333 Seventh Avenue, New York, NY 10001 USA
+1 800 782 3488, customerservice@thieme.com

Thieme Publishers Delhi
A-12, Second Floor, Sector-2, Noida-201301
Uttar Pradesh, India
+91 120 45 566 00, customerservice@thieme.in

Thieme Publishers Rio, Thieme Publicações Ltda.
Edificio Rodolpho de Paoli, 25º andar
Av. Nilo Peçanha, 50 - Sala 2508
Rio de Janeiro 20020-906 Brasil
+55 21 3172 2297 / +55 21 3172 1896

Cover design: Thieme Publishing Group
Cover illustration: Matterhorn image, ©Fotolia,
Aslan Topcu
Typesetting by DiTech Process Solutions, India
Printed in the United States of America
by Publishers' Graphics

ISBN 978-3-13-241279-8   23456

Also available as an e-book:
eISBN 978-3-13-241399-3

Important note: Medicine is an ever-changing science undergoing continual development. Research and clinical experience are continually expanding our knowledge, in particular our knowledge of proper treatment and drug therapy. Insofar as this book mentions any dosage or application, readers may rest assured that the authors, editors, and publishers have made every effort to ensure that such references are in accordance with **the state of knowledge at the time of production of the book**.

Nevertheless, this does not involve, imply, or express any guarantee or responsibility on the part of the publishers in respect to any dosage instructions and forms of applications stated in the book. **Every user is requested to examine carefully** the manufacturers' leaflets accompanying each drug and to check, if necessary in consultation with a physician or specialist, whether the dosage schedules mentioned therein or the contraindications stated by the manufacturers differ from the statements made in the present book. Such examination is particularly important with drugs that are either rarely used or have been newly released on the market. Every dosage schedule or every form of application used is entirely at the user's own risk and responsibility. The authors and publishers request every user to report to the publishers any discrepancies or inaccuracies noticed. If errors in this work are found after publication, errata will be posted at www.thieme.com on the product description page.

Some of the product names, patents, and registered designs referred to in this book are in fact registered trademarks or proprietary names even though specific reference to this fact is not always made in the text. Therefore, the appearance of a name without designation as proprietary is not to be construed as a representation by the publisher that it is in the public domain.

This book is dedicated to Stefa Folke-Sabel, love of my life.

Contents

Preface

Learning and practicing medicine is very time and actually life consuming. In this complex profession a high level of organizational skills is needed to perform your daily duties. Time will become very precious and you will need to become a master of your time: an expert manager of time. However, even perfect organizational skills will not help you to reach goals if you have not defined where you want to go, how you want to live your life and what is important for you. So there is a need for life management as well. With this first edition of *Time & Life Management for Medical Students and Residents* I address what typical medical textbooks do not teach: how to become efficient in the micromanagement of your daily routine and how to keep the perspective of your life as a whole. It is amazing how efficient some of the young residents manage their workload and have a fulfilled and happy life outside the hospital. Unfortunately these guys are pretty rare. It is much more common to see highly motivated residents crash or underperform: in their professional and private life. After 20 years of involvement in Resident training programs I strongly believe that most of the catastrophes could have been prevented and that most of us would benefit from some structural education in time and life management. I hope that this small book helps you to improve your quality of life (and as you are a physician) ultimately also the well-being of your patients as well.

Michael Sabel

Acknowledgment

I would like to thank all participants of the "Time management courses" who helped me with their feedback. Thanks to Frank Willie Floeth MD, PhD and Marion Rapp MD, PhD, best time manager ever.

Introduction

When you start your residency, your life will change dramatically. You will suddenly find yourself in a whirlwind of obligations. Tasks that you have not mastered will be pressed upon you. You will be afraid to fail and you will fail. You will be responsible for complications. Pressure will be incredible, and you will be happy if the day (or quite often the night) is over and you are out of the danger zones. This is how the majority of residents describe their first years and … this is all completely unnecessary. Instead of enjoying your privilege to learn in an elite unit, instead of being proud to make progress in your professional and private life and reaching your goals, and instead of actually enjoying this wonderful job, you sink in a maelstrom of unorganized and chaotic environment. You may feel like you are drowning; here is how you can learn to swim.

A little melodramatic? Yes, but during the last decades nobody cared too much about your situation. Survival of the fittest, publish or perish, and so on are the accepted rules of a medical education. This might be acceptable. However, it is hard to accept that despite hard work, dedicated and motivated residents still fail with catastrophic impact on a whole life. This is especially hard to accept when this is due to wrong planning and thus could have been prevented. I believe it is time for at least a little concern about wasted working hours, inefficiency, and loss of quality of life in young and bright physicians—for the sake of you, the patient, and the rest.

Michael Sabel

About the Book

This book will follow a *macro* to *micro* approach. Let us start with a simple and very schematic model of your life. Figure your life as a journey from A to B. Point A (starting point): now, your actual situation. Point B (destination) is the best possible outcome of your life as a whole.

To reach B you will have to succeed in reaching multiple destinations (**Fig. i** i.e. standing on top of a mountain, becoming chairman etc.). B (best possible outcome of your life as a whole) is the sum of successfully reaching multiple destinations (**Fig. ii**). Note that the "destinations" are defined by time (x-axis) and effort

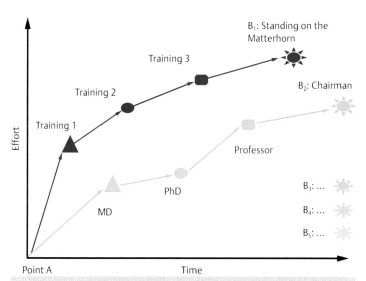

Fig. i To reach goals you need to invest time (x-axis) and effort (y-axis). Before reaching your final goal you need to define sub-goals that are also defined by time and effort as well and need to come in a defined sequence (PhD before Professor, training level 1 before level 2).

$$B = \Sigma \quad {\scriptstyle B_1 + B_2 + B}$$

Fig. ii B (the best possible outcome of your life) is the sum of reaching multiple goals (B1-B...) all defined by time and effort.

(y-axis). The outcome of your life is therefore (among multiple other factors) directly dependent on time and effort. Please keep this simple model in mind when you read the following pages.

- We start with an eagle's perspective (*Part 1: Macro*): from this macro position, it is quite easy to appreciate the roads and destinations (Chapter 1) of your life. Are these the right destinations that you are traveling to? Do you really want to go there? Do you need to go there? We will reflect on the feasibility of your travel logistics (are you physically and mentally capable to reach this goal?).

- Unfortunately, as you have multiple goals (according to your different roles, Chapter 2, **Fig. i**), you are simultaneously traveling in different cars under different conditions in different directions. Some sorting appreciated?

- Do you miss some goals? Have you identified everything on your travel plan that allows you to reach Point B (Chapter 1)?

- If you do not refuel your car and do not maintain it in good shape, you will eventually stop traveling. If you do not eat or drink, you will crash: we will look into regeneration (Chapter 3).

- Now we will start to zoom in (*Part 2: Micro*): we will plan your trip and look into constructing a detailed roadmap. What is the first step? What are the intermediate destinations (Chapter 4)?

- Now we will zoom in even more: you are traveling in different cars with very different levels of complications:

some cars are running by themselves, others are incredibly complicated and need continuous maintenance. Some need to be pushed—to cope with all this, you need to become very efficient (Chapter 5).

- Once you have sorted your stuff, you need to plan and time the performance of pending actions. Therefore, you need to put these into a time frame (Chapter 6).
- Shit will happen. Some advice regarding disaster management (Chapter 7).
- Cope with your anxiety: do not worry, be happy (Chapter 8).
- Are you still on your way? Did you miss an exit? You constantly need to reevaluate your roadmap: so back into the eagle's perspective (Chapter 11).

The general principle of this book's approach is nicely illustrated by a situation, which is usually told on these classical time management seminars. Imagine that you are approached to construct a road in a jungle. Your end points are to do this as cost-effective and fast as possible. You start. With very strong efforts (that make you neglect all other obligations in your life), you become more efficient by the day. The road is rapidly built, and sets new standard in quality and cost efficiency. You feel that you are very successful and on your way. Wrong! You did not check the direction and are about to reach the wrong city. So, what looked like an incredible success becomes a complete failure and worst of all at a very high price. Because you neglected your other obligations, your wife asks for a divorce, you gained 10 kg, there are about 1,000 unanswered e-mails in your account, etc.

Set the right goals, reach these goals efficiently, and adapt the whole system as your situation changes. I hope this book can help you with this endeavor, which is basically to successfully plan the life you want to live.

Part 1 The Eagle's Perspective—"Macro"

During your daily routine you are immersed in multiple obligations that make you virtually blind to the bigger scheme of things. Let us start to look at your life from a superior position that omits the details and gives you a good strategic overview about the roads you are traveling on and the destinations you are going to. This eagle's perspective will help you evaluate your current position in the context of your obligations and adjust and define new goals.

1 Goals

1.1
Importance of Having Goals

Imagine that you are sitting in a small boat. It is stormy, it is raining, and it is cold. Your boat (your position) is subject to waves, wind, and current. This is altogether an unpleasant situation that you want to change. You start to row: initially you are not used to the movement, but with time you are improving—you concentrate on every stroke and eventually you become an efficient rower. After some time, you start to get tired; finally, you have to stop because you are exhausted. You suddenly become aware of your surroundings: the storm is getting worse, it is even more unpleasant than before, and you realize that you are very far away from the land. Thus, despite your (per se *efficient*) efforts to improve your situation and your *motivation* (you pushed yourself to complete exhaustion), your situation is even worse now. Had you applied your rowing skills in the right direction (thus had defined a *goal* before starting to work out like mad), you would be safe and sound on stable ground.

Ideally:
- You would have defined your goal before jumping into action.
- You would have performed efficiently.
- You would have self-regenerated during your journey.

I think it is already obvious from this simple example that you need to define your goal first. I also introduced other important concepts: *motivation*, *efficacy*, and *regeneration*. Do you agree that they are secondary to defining goals? So let us work on goals first.

1.2

Brainstorming Your Goals

Let me stress the importance of goals again. As shown in the example with the jungle road and the rowing boat "incidence," being highly motivated and very efficient in performing is completely useless (and you will still be a loser) if:

- You have no defined goals.
- You have defined the wrong goals (which maybe even worse and very dangerous), that is, unrealistic, too ambitious, too understated, and so on.

We can safely assume that you have goals in your life. It is, however, amazing that many people do not consciously work on this very central hit list of their life.

Are *you* completely aware of your goals?

Exercise 1

Let us do a little exercise, which is the classical opener in many time management courses. Imagine a day in 5 years. You are watching your own funeral. You are listening to your eulogies (for the moment we are focusing on your professional life). So listen to your boss, your colleagues, your patients, etc., talking about your achievements from their different point of views. Let us assume that they are very honest. Now, what will you most likely hear from your boss? What will you hear from your buddies in the hospital? What will you hear from your patients?

Write it down. You will (by proxy) end up with a list of your goals that you (extrapolating your actual situation) might have achieved. Are you surprised? Disappointed? Were you immediately aware of these goals? Or did you have to think hard before you were able to write down one of the essential list of your life? Did you just realize that you defined goals which were defined a couple of years ago? Are they still valid?

Exercise 2

Let Exercise 1 settle down for a little time. Now you take the direct approach: define where you want to stand in 5 years (again, for the moment we are focusing on your professional life). Be as precise as possible—instead of projecting that you will do neuro-surgery, define the date of your board examination ("in 5 years I will prepare for the board, which I will sit in September 2018"), I will have specialized in neuro-oncology with more than 300 procedures as leading surgeon, I will have finished my PhD thesis (title?), I will have published 30 peer-reviewed papers, etc.

You get the point. This is not a project you can do in 5 minutes. If you really want to take advantage of these exercises, invest time.

1.3
Mechanics of Success

As a result of Exercises 1 and 2, you will now have brand new goals at your hands. I suspect that you are very eager to start on your journey to reach the goal(s). However, the decision to go for a goal is a very important decision and can have huge consequences on virtually all aspects of your life. It is therefore almost essential to understand the underlying mechanisms, which determine your success or failure. Before jumping in, put your goal to a reality check.

1.4

The "You Can Make It If You Want" Nonsense

The difficulty in choosing a goal is to avoid underestimation of your capabilities. On the other hand, overestimation is problematic as well. A huge part of success and motivation literature is filled with witty little statements such as: *you can make it if you really want*. No, actually you cannot, if you choose to run a marathon under 2.03 hours or plan to become a commercial pilot with poor eyesight. Therefore, perform a reality check by evaluation of the available logistics of your life.

In a schematic drawing (**Fig. 1.1**), I set your goal in the context of a timeline (x-axis) and work required (y-axis). This simple

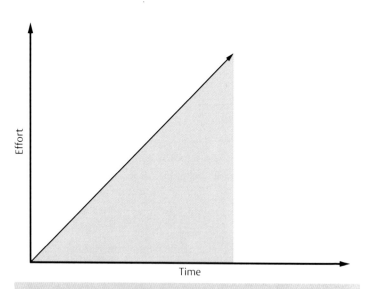

Fig. 1.1 This "mechanical" model describes that you need to invest time and effort to reach a goal. The "area under the curve" represents the energy that you need to spend and is dependent on the time and effort needed to reach your goal.

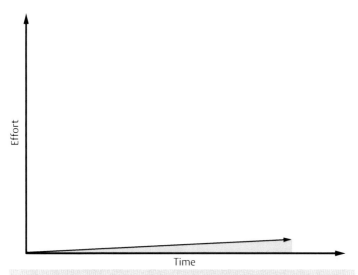

Fig. 1.2 Here the energy needed to reach your goal is much less than in Fig. 1.1: you decided to reach a goal that requires lesser effort and you have decided to reach it much later.

model shows that you need to invest work to reach your goal: the more ambitious your goal, the more work you need to invest. Note that the position of your goal is also within a time frame. The shorter time you plan to reach your goal and the more ambitious your goal is, the more *energy* you need to invest (area under the curve). If you plan to reach a less ambitious goal in a longer time period you will need to invest lesser energy (**Fig. 1.2**).

Another important point: if you have reached your goal, you have (according to our rather crude mechanical model) acquired a certain potential energy (**Fig. 1.3**). In terms of physics, there are two consequences:

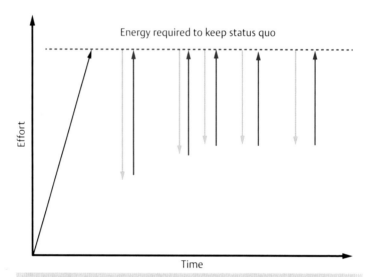

Fig. 1.3 The higher you climb, the deeper you fall, and, according to this simple model, you need to invest energy to stay on the level you reached.

1. You need to spend energy to stay on this level.
2. If you do not, you will fall. The higher you climbed, the deeper you will fall.

2 Roles

Up to this point, we have focused on just one (professional) aspect of your life and have considered only one goal. *First*, you will need to define more than one goal in your professional life and, *second*, you are involved in multiple jobs, for which you have to define multiple goals.

Apart from being a neurosurgeon, with your freshly defined goal to publish 12 papers in the next 19 months, you might also be a father, a husband, an ambitious soccer player, a cook, etc. The point is you need to consider your professional goal in the context of multiple other goals. In social sciences, these multiple jobs you are involved in are called *roles*.

2.1
Identify Your Roles

From a certain point of view, everything you are is defined by your roles. Roles define where you are and what you are supposed to do; they are directly correlated with your success. They determine your quality of life.

Exercises 3 and 4

Sit down and try to identify all the roles (professional and private) that you are engaged in.

Professionally, you may be a senior resident (physician), you may be in charge of an educational program for younger residents (teacher), you may be the speaker of residents (politician), you may have a research project (scientist), etc. In your private life, you might be a spouse, mother/father, lover, friend, cook, athlete, hobby artist, dog owner, chairman of your local charity club, etc. It needs only a little brainstorming to come up with a list (Exercise 4).

- Physician
- Scientist
- Teacher
- Hobby cook
- Mother/father
- Athlete, etc.

Look at the list. You might be amazed in how many roles you are already involved. Are you happy with all these roles? Do you want to get rid of some? Are there roles that you want to play but you are not yet involved in? Start to sort your roles in an order of importance.

This is a very important and in principle very simple sorting process. In reality, however, this is very difficult: is your residency more important than being a husband/father (classical conflict)? Be honest to yourself.

2.2
Your Social Position as Defined by Roles and Goals

Now, as you have this snapshot of your social position in your hand, the next step is to go back to Chapter 1 and define the goals for each role (Exercise 4). Take a year off for this. Now your actual social position is more likely described by **Fig. 2.1**.

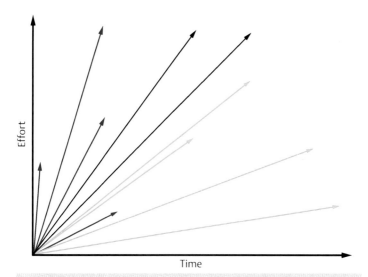

Fig. 2.1 Your actual position in life: you want to reach multiple goals with different time frames and levels of efforts.

2.3

Reinvent Yourself

Of course, you will most likely not take a year off for this, but believe me there are many less important thing that you could do for yourself in a year's time. Understand that you can put yourself in a position where you stand at the drawing board of your life. You can reinvent yourself. During this process you will get rid of some goals, and you will have redefined old and defined new goals. You might also have to cancel and refine new roles. And as the sum of your roles defines your life, you need to consider the balance of your roles as a whole.

If you take this suggestion seriously, you will have the chance to reconfirm your goals, redefine your life, and think a lot about very important issues that you have neglected.

However, there are some severe drawbacks: as we have discussed before, every goal has an area under the curve. This is the energy that you have to invest to reach the goal. The height that you reach implements that you need to continuously spend energy to stay at that level. If you have to spend 54 hours per week in the hospital, how realistic is a training program that puts you 10 hours per week on a bike? How much time is left for your partner? How much time is left for your children, your dog, and your friends? How much time for yourself?

And time is not the only issue: it is energy that you need to spend. As you well know, your energy is not inexhaustible. You need to invest it cautiously, avoiding unnecessary frictions and losses, due to organizational and logistic problems.

So several new issues are coming up: regeneration, efficiency, prioritization, and organization. We will start with regeneration.

3 Regeneration

> *"If I had to spend 6 hours to chop down a tree, I would spend the first hour to sharpen the axe."*
>
> Abraham Lincoln

Imagine you are traveling in a car. You are very eager to reach your destination. You are focused and you are making good time. However, your wife points out that the car is running out of fuel and suggests that you stop to gas up. You respond: "I do not have time for this." This will spare you about 5 minutes, but in the end this could completely destroy your end point.

An example from Stephen Covey's legendary book *The 7 Habits of Highly Effective People* puts it nicely to the point:

> You observe a man who is trying to saw down a tree. He is working very hard but makes only little progress. You ask him if he's all right and he answers that he is at his limits and almost completely exhausted. You suggest that he takes a break and sharpens the saw. His response: "I don't have time to sharpen the saw. I am too busy sawing ...."

These little examples illustrate how self-destructive our work habits can become. You want to be as productive as possible, but in the attempt to reach your goal you are destroying your productivity. Almost everyone is familiar with Aesop's fable, "The Goose That Laid the Golden Eggs" (Perry index 70). Killing the goose that laid the golden eggs is a good example for an action motivated by greed that eventually destroys the productivity and thus the profit.

If you are too greedy to regenerate, you will destroy your productivity.

Practicing medicine is a very long and difficult journey. Combining this ambitious goal with all the other aspects of your life is very demanding. To reach your destination (point B, About the Book), you will need to continuously regenerate the most important tool that you have: yourself.

Obviously, this is not only concerning your body, though physical fitness and health are of utmost importance. This is also very much concerning your mind.

Traditionally, philosophers describe four dimensions of the human nature that need constant care and active reevaluation and regeneration: physical, spiritual, mental, and social/emotional.

3.1
Physical

As you are a physician, we will not go into the detailed background of sports medicine. However, consider some practical suggestions. As you enter your residency program, your time schedule fundamentally changes. The first thing that you might consider to skip is physical activity. You simply do not have the time. Believe me: you can overcome many of the work-induced restraints, at least regarding simple workout plans (if you used to spent 5 hours on a golf course I am not so sure) by adaptation. Due to the fitness boom, gyms are virtually everywhere (how many on your way to the hospital?), some are open 24/7, most of these at least until 10 PM. Consider to end your day by passing by; 30 minutes with the right training are fine. Apart from the physical benefits, this is an efficient way to decompress. Or how about taking the bicycle to work or running?

Since Mark Lauren has popularized the concept of body weight training, you have always access to a very effective whole body training, which you can easily perform in your office.

Most of the residents are on a strange diet—a cup of coffee in the morning and several more during the day, and with growing appetite during the day, they start to eat virtually everything that is available on the wards. This ends up in the consumption of mountains of sweets and cakes topped off with ordering a pizza at home or at work. Caffeine-free water intake is usually below 500 mL. If a physician would take this diet as a history from a patient, he would shake his head and advise an appointment with a nutritionist.

All this might be a little exaggerated, but you will certainly recognize the problem. Taking care of your diet is very important. You absolutely must not be hungry or thirsty during work! You need to drink at least 2 L of water during working hours (8 hours). Make sure that water is available and make sure that you have consumed it. Put eight marks on the bottle, one for each hour, and check your drinking pattern. Consider bringing your food to the hospital. A sandwich prepared at home, fruits, or the leftover from dinner is always better than consuming the empty carbohydrates on the wards.

Prepare a proper dinner. Since supermarkets are open until late, there is no excuse for having an empty fridge. There is no need for lengthy cooking. Since Jamie Oliver and Nigella Lawson have published their apps fresh, healthy and very tasty food can be prepared by everyone in less than 20 minutes. As the recipes come with electronic shopping lists and detailed description how to prepare the meal (again: 20 minutes max), there is no need for fast food consumption at all. Prepare a little more and you have your next day's lunch.

As your body is now well fed, water balanced, and fit, we change subject and consider mental dimensions.

3.2
Spiritual

To clarify what I mean with "spiritual," I quote Dr. Puchalski:

> Spirituality is the aspect of humanity that refers to the way individuals seek and express meaning and purpose and the way they experience their connectedness to the moment, to self, to others, to nature, and to the significant or sacred. (Puchalski et al 2009)

I choose this definition of spirituality because it defines the goal of spirituality as the quest for a value system, independent from a specific religiousness.

Revisit your values. The exercise we did in Chapter 1 can help in identifying your values and what you stand for.

Exercise 5

Again, you are watching your own funeral. You are listening to the eulogies, which are addressing the values you stand for and how you lived them. Of course, you need to be very honest to yourself.

As your self-awareness might not be objective enough, you might consider asking a trusted person with intimate knowledge of your personality to listen to your self-evaluation.

I strongly suggest that you repeatedly perform an examination of your motives. Examine your value system. Who are you? What is your definition of good? Are you (at present) living according to your values? Are the changes that you are going to implement consistent with your inner values? Are you making moral compromises?

The classical questions you should ask yourself are:

If you would meet yourself, would you like this person? If you are your spouse, would you still be in love? Would you still be your friend? Why would anyone like you, be in love with you, respect you, trust you? Hopefully, you will come up with answers like: because I have a nice humor, because I am gentle, sensitive, I am good at what I am doing, etc.

This is a very difficult exercise, which is per se never objective. Hence, there is a need for external evaluation. Try to get this by having yourself evaluated by your friends, spouse, and family. In your professional life, you should have evaluation talks at some checkpoints anyway.

3.3
Mental

After formal education, most of us abandon any education outside our field of professional focus. We slowly develop into nerds. This is, of course, unfortunate. The result is a degeneration of our intellect and the incapability of intellectual development and growth. Continuing your education is important. You need to expose your intellect to challenges very different from your professional focus. Reading books, visits to a theater, museums, or cinema: pick your poison. Reading Ulysses at the end of a working day will overstrain most of us. The important point is, however, not the intellectual level of the challenge: it is the stimulation of your mind, the exploration of the yet unknown, and your evaluation of its values. This is probably very different for different personalities. To be very honest, when I decided to regularly attend visits to our theater I was not so impressed. No challenge. No self-renewal. No new insights. When my cousin Martin, however, introduced me to our local soccer club, I was thrilled. As I was never interested in soccer, this was something new, a very different social environment with very different rules. So, Fortuna Düsseldorf regenerates my value system and keeps it up to date.

3.4
Social/Emotional

For most of us, it will be quite obvious that a functional social and emotional life is of utmost importance for our well-being. You need a partner you can trust, with whom you can decompress. You need love and sex. You need friends. You need their crucial feedback regarding your values and you need their new impulses. You need parties. For many of us, at least a little "Sex and drugs and Rock n Roll" is part of our social culture.

Unfortunately, all these aspects are at high risk because of your professional life. When you return from 12 hours intense verbal interaction with patients and colleagues, how many words are left for your spouse or your children? Do have the energy to pick up the phone and call your mother or your friends? Don't you rather enjoy a relaxing mutism? You will often feel that you have overdrawn your lexical budget for the day.

Typical situation at 8 PM

Spouse: "How was your day in the hospital, darling?"
Resident: "Grunt. What's for dinner?"

If that is the end of your social interaction for that evening, your relationship has a worse prognosis than any cancer patient you have seen that day.

On the other hand, you just do not feel like talking in this moment, you just cannot. It does not help your relationship if you need to steal yourself for a forced communication after work. What you need to do is to realize and accept this job-induced handicap. There are very practical solutions for this (see Part 2). But, first, realize the problem.

An interesting aspect of residency is that you are exposed to and involved in rather dramatic aspects of life. You are a protagonist in *ER or Gray's Anatomy*. You are in the center of the attention of your patients. The relatives hang on your lips; you are very important. You make crucial life and death decisions. You have tremendous success. You fail. And then you are just a mother, a father, a friend, or a spouse. You are forced to strip off your superheroes' costume and return to the normal life. Coming home, you will have to listen to the tiny, little, banal, and unimportant problems your partner or friends have suffered through. You see the problem? If you do not accept that these problems are as important as yours and if you are not able to listen, you will have a fundamental problem in your social relationships.

It does not help your social interactions that in most residency programs your position is within a military hierarchy. This is pretty unique. You are part of a clear chain of command. That changes when you leave the hospital.

Unfortunately, it will not be sufficient to excel in only one of the four dimensions. One of the crucial problems that you need to solve is to find a functional balance between the four dimensions: physical, spiritual, mental, and social/emotional (**Fig. 3.1**).

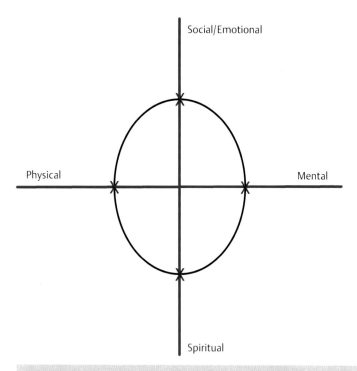

Fig. 3.1 Using this diagram, you can evaluate your balance between the four dimensions: physical, spiritual, mental, and social/emotional: just put a cross where you (obviously subjectively) believe your actual position regarding these dimensions is located. Though it is unclear which configuration is ideal (a perfect circle?), it helps you to visualize imbalances.

Intermezzo: You are the boss (of your life)

Before we change from the macroscopic view into the microscopic view, thus before we change from strategic decision-making to micromanagement, there is one important aspect of your life that you need to have always available in your mind.

You Are the Boss (of Your Life)

If you stop reading this and return to your social interactions, you will be under siege. Everybody is pounding you with demands, you receive orders, you are obliged to function, you are chained into a confusing amount of obligations, etc. You are suffocating.

There is a very important axiom of our social life.

> You are in command of yourself. You have always the choice to get out of the situation.
>   Always and immediately.

If you absolutely need to, just walk out. Of course, there are consequences, but this is not the point here. You need to keep this in your mind: ultimately you decide about your life. Do not see yourself as a passive victim: you are the boss.

From Stimulus to Response

Between stimulus and response there is a space. In that space is our power to choose our response. In our response lies our growth and our freedom.

Viktor E. Frankl

The space that Frankl describes is the difference between animal and human. It is the space in which you decide how to react to a demand from your superior, how you respond to the suffering of a patient, to aggressive behavior, or positive emotions. Read Frankl in more depth and you will understand that it is not our actual crisis that is hurting us, but our response to it. In our, on a first glance, very heteronomous life, we *always* have our personal freedom to decide how to react on a stimulus.

Part 2 Boots on the Ground—"Micro"

Allow me to come back to the travel paradigm from the introduction. Up to now, we have worked on the road map. You now have very clear ideas about your destinations, and you are sure they are the right ones and that they will ultimately carry you to point B. All you need is to start. And here most of us stop. There is a big difference and a long way to go between elaborated goal and actual action.

4 From Goal to Action

4.1
Procrastination

One of the big problems we usually confront when we make the transition from plan to action is that we avoid starting. We want to avoid the unpleasant workload that is ahead of us. We often fall into the habit of "procrastination," thus avoid doing a task that needs to be accomplished. There are usually two correlated reasons for this behavior:

- Lack of motivation (remember when you postponed to study until the night before the exam?).
- The inertness to start, because you have no idea how to start.

Let us skip from the car-driving paradigm to mountain climbing. Imagine that you are in principle capable to perform complicated rock climbing. After lecture of Part 1 of this book, you have decided that one of the important goals of your life is to climb the Matterhorn (**Fig. 4.1**). Just looking at this mountain might intimidate most of us and induce a severe bout of procrastination: "this is not manageable, not today, maybe tomorrow, I have an urgent appointment with my coiffeur and so on ...." If this project is not really important for you, then walk away from it: no harm done. However, if the project is important, then you are in big trouble by walking away. The urge to accomplish and to deliver will catch up with you and will add to the many nagging voices in your subconsciousness. Eventually, the pressure might become so overwhelming that you start climbing. There are several drawbacks with this procedure. First, you went through a tough time with the nagging

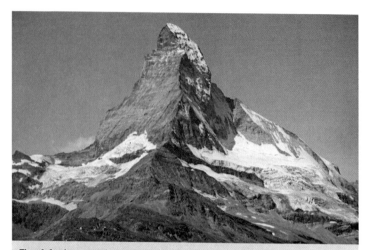

Fig. 4.1 The Matterhorn as an example for a goal: beautiful but very intimidating. Impossible to reach the top?

voice constantly accusing you of your insufficiency. Second, your pressure-generated motivation might make you blind for weather problems and you are climbing under less than optimal conditions.

4.2
The Stepwise Approach

A very efficient way to overcome this "procrastination problem" is to transfer this huge, monstrous project into manageable portions (actions). **Fig. 4.2** shows you the subdivision of this monster climb into manageable steps (at least for the few mountain climber capable to do this), so that your perspective is a now and

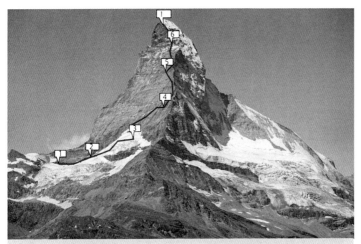

Fig. 4.2 By planning small steps, this monster goal is divided into manageable steps.

immediately manageable action (**Fig. 4.3**). Therefore, after defining a goal, you need to sit down and define the subsequent steps that you need to make (**Fig. 4.4**). This is a crucial point. You need to translate the goal into manageable steps (= actions).

4.3

The Need to Define the First Action

Take extra care to design an easy first action. Once you have started, things often become easier and are carried by the momentum that develops after successfully climbing the first step.

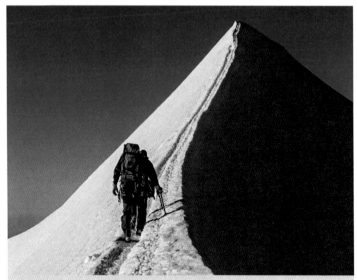

Fig. 4.3 A manageable step: just a few hundred meters and you have completed the planned action.

Forward and Backward Organization

By subdividing a complex problem into manageable steps/actions, it is essential that you:

- Identify all necessary actions.
- Put them in the right sequence.

One of the very effective ways to do this is to walk through a timeline. It is often useful to start with the end point. Imagine that you organize a meeting. Think at the closing session. What is needed at this point? Brainstorm the actions that come in mind:

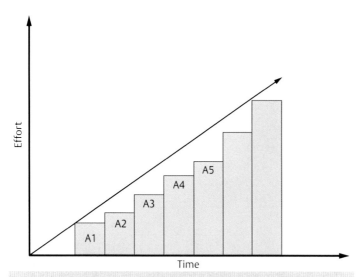

Fig. 4.4 Sequence of actions needed to reach the goal. In most cases, you will need to plan a specific sequence; in contrast to the graph shown here, there is not necessarily an increasing amount of effort needed.

flowers for the organizers, certifications, in which location, date of next meeting, transfers to the airport, time the meeting stops, time for the transfers, etc. Note all the actions that come in mind and repeat that exercise with a forward approach. You will end up with long list of items (actions). Now sort them into a logical sequence: according to time frame, importance, etc.

Exercise 6

Choose one of your goals and start "sequencing."

5 Sorting

The Need to Triage

As a result of Exercise 6 and your further application of this approach to the hopefully multiple goals, you now have identified a myriad of pending actions, which you need to accomplish to reach point B. Now (Exercise 7, **Fig. 5.1**), imagine your next working day and list the routine actions that you will need to deal with, add the potential additional actions due to emergency cases, and proceed by listing actions that need to be done by the end of next week and end of the month. No, you are not finished yet: add to the list all the

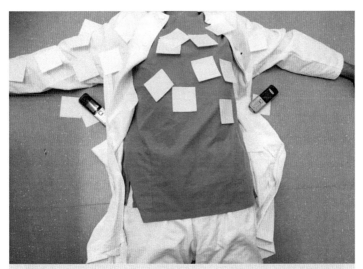

Fig. 5.1 Killed by exploded inbox.

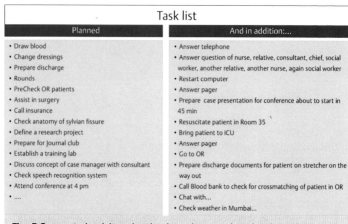

Task list	
Planned	**And in addition:...**

• Draw blood
• Change dressings
• Prepare discharge
• Rounds
• PreCheck OR patients
• Assist in surgery
• Call insurance
• Check anatomy of sylvian fissure
• Define a research project
• Prepare for Journal club
• Establish a training lab
• Discuss concept of case manager with consultant
• Check speech recognition system
• Attend conference at 4 pm
• ....
	• Answer telephone
	• Answer question of nurse, relative, consultant, chief, social
	  worker, another relative, another nurse, again social worker
	• Restart computer
	• Answer pager
	• Prepare case presentation for conference about to start in
	  45 min
	• Resuscitate patient in Room 35
	• Bring patient to ICU
	• Answer pager
	• Go to OR
	• Prepare discharge documents for patient on stretcher on the
	  way out
	• Call Blood bank to check for crossmatching of patient in OR
	• Chat with...
	• Check weather in Mumbai...

Fig. 5.2 A typical task list. Already a busy day regarding the planned actions. "And in addition ..." will probably kill your day.

actions that you need to accomplish in your private life. Look at the bright side of this: you are in high demand. On the other hand, you are probably on the verge of a nervous breakdown. Many persons might decompress under this workload of actions and will freeze (**Fig. 5.2**). Others will start to work. They jump into activity and accomplish actions that need immediate attention. These are usually the actions labeled urgent. This is in principle a very honorable approach. However, there is an inherent risk that these persons will never find the time to tackle the actions necessary to reach one of their important goals. The actions necessary for important goals are not urgent, only important. Go back to the list of actions you will probably need to perform tomorrow. Ask yourself which of the listed actions will most likely influence your position in 10 years (**Fig. 5.2**). Unfortunately, most of the actions will have no impact at all (apart from the fact that neglect of some of these will get you in deep trouble). In the end, a triage based on urgency alone will let you cope with the moment, and the day and the week. But that is it. You waste your energy and your future in daily firefighting. And, while you are putting out fires, you are inadvertently covering the back of someone who has time to work on his goals. What you need is an intelligent triage system. I recommend President Eisenhower:

> I have two kinds of problems: the urgent and the important. The urgent are not important, and the important are never urgent. (Dwight D. Eisenhower 1954)

The principle of this approach is to decide if the pending action is urgent or important or urgent and important or neither urgent nor important.

5.2
Time Matrix/Eisenhower's Principle

Covey labeled the four Eisenhower categories "Quadrants" and introduced the *time matrix* (**Fig. 5.3**):

- Quadrant I (QI; top left) contains important, urgent items—items that need to be dealt with immediately.
- Quadrant II (QII; top right) contains important, but not urgent items—items that are important but do not require your immediate attention. This is the quadrant that includes the necessary actions for your long-term goals.
- In Quadrant III (QIII; bottom left), we have urgent, but unimportant items—items that should be minimized or eliminated. These are the time sucks, the "poor planning on your part does not constitute an emergency on my part" variety of tasks.

	Urgent	Not Urgent
Important	I • Crises • Pressing problems • Firefighting • Major scrap and rework • Deadline-driven projects	II • Prevention • Production capability activities • Relationship building • Recognizing new opportunities • Planning • Re-creation
Not Important	III • Interruptions • Some calls • Some mail • Some reports • Some meetings • Proximate pressing matters • Popular activities • Some scrap & rework	IV • Trivia • Busy work • Some mail • Some phone calls • Time-wasters • Pleasant activities

Fig. 5.3 The time matrix, a simple but very important (and effective way) to sort your inbox. Focus on quadrant II.

- Quadrant IV (QIV; bottom right) contains unimportant and also not urgent items—items that do not have to be done anytime soon, perhaps add little to no value, and should be minimized or eliminated. These are often trivial time wasters.

The next exercise is obvious?!

Exercise 8

Sort all the actions that you have identified in Exercise 7 into the four quadrants. This is a typical QII action: very important but not urgent.

Sorting your actions is, however, only the first step and constitutes only the essential basis for a much more important step: you need to organize your life in way that you spent as much (working) time as possible in QII, avoid QIV, delegate QIII, and keep QI as small as possible. This sounds quite simple but putting this into practice might require severe changes of your behavior in your professional and private life. You probably need to change your attitude toward your colleagues, your work, your superiors, and subordinates. To clarify the impact of spending time in the wrong quadrant, I will elaborate the quadrants a little more in detail.

5.3

QI

You will not be able to avoid QI (urgent and important). It contains the emergencies and the crises. Of course, you will not walk away from a CPR, because you need to write an outline of your PhD thesis (QII). You will probably pick up a ringing telephone or answer your pager, despite working on a paper (QII). Staying in QI is easy, because you do not have to plan: you just react. And with growing skills you will feel more and more comfortable with the actions thrown at you, because you will master the CPR and the telephone call might even relieve you from working on a difficult intellectual problem. However, as long as you focus on QI, this quadrant will become larger and larger until you will be buried and consumed by emergency actions thrown at you (**Fig. 5.1**). One of the natural consequences of this overload is that you escape into QIV (not urgent/not important) to relax. You play a game, chat with a colleague, check the weather on the weekend, etc. This might help you to decompress, but does not help to change your need to stay in QI. You live a life dominated by crisis. This might be intense but at the end you will not have achieved any of your very important goals. They happen in QII.

5.4
QIII

Depending on your experience, you might believe that you are working in QI, but it is actually QIII (urgent/not important). Typically, the urgency of the actions is based on the priorities and expectations of others. These are the actions you need to decline or delegate. A typical example is a ringing phone (urgent, might be important). As you pick up, you have a request for an appointment in 3 months (urgent/not important): something you need to delegate to your secretary ASAP, so that you can return to work on your thesis (QII).

5.5
QII

QII is the heart of effective personal management. Here are the actions you need to accomplish to reach your goals. The inherent problem of these actions is that they are not urgent, so you do not get around to getting them done. Or they will be forgotten and your goal will not be reached, or they will become urgent and important and add to your QI problem. Typical example: you are invited to give a lecture in 3 months. It is an *important* lecture. Given that you have 3 months' time, it is *not urgent* (QII). You plan to introduce new slights and data (actions) in an already existing ppt. You estimate that you need 6-hour total working time. Instead of planning to work on the presentation in an elective mode (sit down for 1 hour every week), you procrastinate and oops: the talk is next week and nothing has been done so far. The shift of these actions into QI will probably influence the quality of the presentation, will influence your management of other QI activities, and will greatly add to your anxiety level. The more time you spent in QII, the smaller QI will become. As a consequence, you will have more time for QII, which further decreases QI. Finally, a positive vicious circle is created.

The sorting of your pending actions by the *time matrix* approach has provided you with a very important tool: an efficient strategy. However, this is an intellectual concept only. What you need to do now is to put it into practice.

It is 7 AM, Monday morning. You are on the ward. Deliver. You need to execute 1,000 actions.

5.6
Execute Actions

Now we further zoom in, we are on the ground. You are on rounds, the telephone is ringing, the OR is waiting, you need to present a patient on grand rounds tomorrow, you have at least 60 unanswered e-mails in your inbox, you need to buy a birthday present, there is a lecture you need to give in 3 weeks, the proofs of a paper need to be returned to the editor by tomorrow, you have to write a discharge letter, and a yet undisclosed number of actions on the ward—in summary, a very normal Monday morning. The least of your problems in your actual situation is QII. This is no elective. This is chaos. Everything is "urgent." You are urged to accomplish as many actions as effectively as possible. Or more specifically:

- You need to evaluate the action. Does it belong to a QI/QIII setting?
- You need to accomplish the actions in the right order (triage).
- You must not forget actions.

The traditional way to deal with this situation is a to-do list.

5.7
To-Do or Not-to-Do

At 7.30, you will end up with a list of several new actions, pending your attention: a to-do list. If it is a classical to-do list, it will be a sheet of paper with several items. These are probably in the order in which they have been presented to you. This list is only an inventory with the only merit that you might not forget actions. These kinds of lists are ineffective and right out dangerous. If you sit down and work through the actions from top to bottom without any sorting, you might reach action no. 12 (patient claims allergy against paracetamol, put note to file) 10 minutes after application of the drug. Obviously, you need to sort these items into QI and QII. You will then have a to-do (now) and a not-to-do (now) list in your hands. Better, but far from perfect. Let us assume that you have five actions with comparable levels of urgency on your to-do (now) list. The first one requires you to draw blood in room 54, the second action requires you to check laboratory values in the computer, the third action is checking the wound in room 55, the fourth action is checking for a pathology report in the PC, and the fifth is to remove drainage in room 55. I will not insult your intelligence, but sticking to the order of your checklist you would quite inefficiently run from patient to PC, PC to patient, and so on. From this simple example, it becomes obvious that a simple to-do list will *not do*.

5.8
The In-Box-Out-Box Approach

Let us analyze your situation at this point. By defining your goals, you identified a large number of rather elective, but nevertheless pending, actions. These are the things you prefer to do (QII).

However, all other quadrants are filled up with actions as well; in fact, you have just spent hours in the "urgent department."

In addition, you will probably sit on a rather huge pile of yet amorphous "stuff" that needs to be processed as well (you have not made it to your inbox in the post office yet, but you have been told that it is full). Despite your epic job performance during the last hours, you feel that there is still an overwhelming workload. There is a gigantic to-do list and a big pile of still unknown stuff waiting for you. All these actions and the unprocessed stuff are nagging in your subconsciousness and making you feel uneasy and irritable.

Take some time off and let us approach the situation systematically. Read through the text below and get the idea. However, before you actually start with the sorting, labeling, and cleaning process, before you create folders and start to work with a calendar, consider engaging dedicated software. You can, of course, use pen, folders, and notebooks. However, I believe that you greatly increase you efficiency and mobility by working with computer, handhelds, and cloud. One of the big advantages is that you have always access to your inbox. Thus, ideas, actions, and new obligations can be deposited there from everywhere and will not get lost.

Let us consider that all demands, tasks, pending actions, and obligations of your professional and private life (in summary, everything you need to do or care for) are accumulated in one virtual inbox (**Fig. 5.4**). In this inbox, everything you need to work on is accumulated. Your job is to process this "stuff" until it can be transferred into the outbox (**Fig. 5.5**). Things that are in your inbox are problems (your problems); things that are in the outbox are solved problems (or problems of other peoples). Hence, your efficiency is greatly dependent on the way you work with your inbox or in other words how you *empty* your inbox.

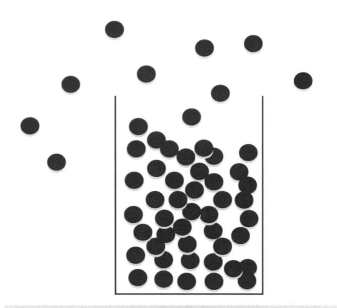

Fig. 5.4 A virtual inbox. Put all the pending actions in this place.

Step 1 (Collection Process)

Go to your office. Take your "inbox." Start with a real box, but have a virtual box (simple word file will do to get the principle idea) available. Fill the real box with the content of your post box and the stuff that is on your desk. Pile everything that is pending into that box. For virtual tasks, write down a note and put it in the inbox (virtual inbox or print it out).

Step 2 (Sorting)

There are several very important ways to approach the overwhelming workload now accumulated in your inbox. You might

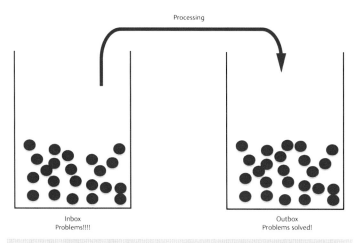

Fig. 5.5 The goal is to empty your inbox by processing the stuff in the inbox to outbox. Every item moved is an immediate problem solved.

do this in one process deciding in parallel decision processes or you might decide to clean your inbox under just one of the following aspects.

5.9

Sorting Your Inbox

Sort the stuff in your inbox into the following categories.

Actions

These are already clearly defined and therefore manageable tasks. As explained earlier, it is very important that you transfer complex tasks into workable items and defined actions (**Fig. 4.4**). The action is your working horse. It is the place where you get your work done.

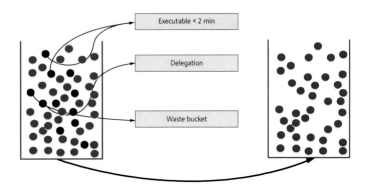

Fig. 5.6 The options you have to transfer items into the outbox.

Examples:
- Call Dr. Kamp (mobile number provided).
- Check laboratory values of patient MS.
- Buy four AAA batteries.
- Insert illustrations into presentation.

Check your inbox for actions. For each action, you need to determine a first *cleaning* step (**Fig. 5.6**).

Executable in Less Than 2 Minutes?

If so, do it now (call Dr. Kamp). If not, proceed as outlined in the following. It makes no sense to spent processing time for actions that can be cleared in less than 2 minutes.

Delegation Yes/No

If yes, action is cleared into the inbox of a colleague. Done.

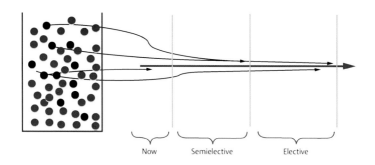

Now   Semielective   Elective

Fig. 5.7 Sorting process according to urgency.

Waste

Easy. Delete. Waste bucket.

For the remaining actions, you need to determine the following.

Timing

Determine a date when this action has to be executed (**Fig. 5.7**). Timeline categories should include the heads: now, semielective and elective. Put it to file with a date. Make sure to use a system that provides a reminder function.

Context

Most of the actions can only be executed under specific conditions. For example, the action "buy four AAA batteries" can only be executed when you are standing in front of a shelf with four AAA batteries (in a shop). Ideally, the action to buy batteries

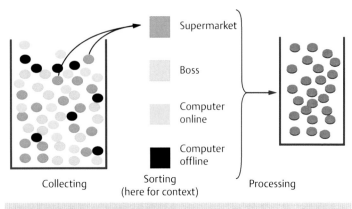

Fig. 5.8 Sorting process according to context.

should engage your mind only in the moment when you are actually standing in front of the right shelf. To this end, you need to label the action with Monday 8 PM and put in a context "supermarket/battery shelf." As you enter the supermarket, you check the context supermarket. You get the point. Consider to use this approach also for people. Imagine that in your inbox are several items that you need to discuss with your boss. Check your file "boss" before entering his office: you have a complete list of things you want to discuss (**Fig. 5.8**).

5.10

Goals

Your goals should be in your (virtual) inbox as well.

If you have followed my suggestions, you would have already defined the necessary actions, which will be processed as described earlier.

If your goal is complex, then I suggest you subdivide the goal in several projects. If your goal is, for example, to finish your PhD thesis, you could establish projects for parts of your work:

Goal: PhD thesis

- Project—discussion of paper
  Action: read paper by Smith on brain plasticity. Due April 1, 2016, 6 PM.
- Project—talk
  Action: insert figures. Due April 12, 2016, 4 PM.
- Project—cooperation with Kamp's laboratory
  Action: call Dr. Kamp (mobile number provided). Due April 1, 2016, 6 PM.

5.11
New Ideas

These are potential goals in statu nascendi and most likely QII relevant. I suggest formulating an action, that is, "consider role of surgery for butterfly glioblastoma." Label it with QII and if necessary with a date for reconsideration and put it in a folder "Ideas."

5.12
Amorphous Stuff

What do you do with a request to review a paper? To join a research project? To attend a conference? To give a talk? You might not be able to decide. Put this in an "Observation/pending decision folder" and establish a date for review of the content.

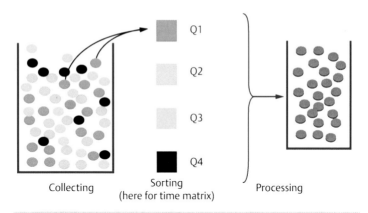

Q1

Q2

Q3

Q4

Collecting   Sorting   Processing
                 (here for time matrix)

Fig. 5.9 Sorting process according to time matrix criteria.

5.13
Trash

Easy.

Time Matrix

Probably the most important way to sort your inbox is the classi-
fication according *time matrix* criteria (**Fig. 5.9**). Sort your inbox
(actions and projects) according to QI–QIV criteria.

At the end of the day, your inbox might not be empty, but most
of the stuff is organized and labeled. Cleaning your inbox should
become a regular QII activity. You have control. You know what to
do (action), when to do (dates), and where to do (context). You know
what is important and what is not. You have a clear idea where strategic import work is waiting. Now you need to make sure that you
have time to work on your important projects. Plan your work.

6   Planning Your Week

As a result of the reading so far, you should have realized that it is essential for you to do on a regular basis things that are very important but not urgent. You need to organize your life in a way that guarantees that:

- You spent as much time as possible in QII.
- You integrate regeneration with the four dimensions: physical, spiritual, mental, and social/emotional.

Unfortunately, our work habits will push us into QI and QIII, thus preventing us from spending time for these essential aspects. They will, however, not prevent you from spending time for an unimportant conference that is scheduled for next week at 4 PM (probably a classical QIII time waster). I suggest that you schedule the four dimensions—physical, spiritual, mental, and social/emotional—and QII activities as you schedule your surgery, lectures, conferences, etc. Plan these activities ahead. Use the time frame of a week. Plan the week in a way that allows for integration of the really important aspect.

Exercise 9

Draw a table or open a spread sheet: 7 columns (=days) and 18 rows (=hours, label the rows beginning at 5 AM through 10 PM). That is your next week. Let us assume, for the sake of convenience, that you work from 7 AM to 5 PM. You are not on call and free on Saturday and Sunday. Now please mark the time slots in which you are probably completely other-directed (use red, please). These are probably the QI and QIII aspects of your working time. These are also the time slots that you must attend rounds, time in the OR, conferences, etc., in which you will not be able to attend to any QII activities. Accept this and do not plan for QII activities in these periods. Now plan your QII activities (within the time frame of 7 AM to 5 PM). Mark time slots (use green, please). As QII requires brain power, consider your biological clock (are you at your best in the morning or afternoon?). Now mark slots (within the time frame of 7 AM to 5 PM) for QI activities (use light gray, please). These are slots reserved for urgent and important actions that you cannot take care of in the "red" periods. Mark slots (within the time frame of 7 AM to 5 PM) for trivia and busy work (use dark gray, please). Use the time slots when you are usually tired and lacking in concentration. Now you start with scheduling your regeneration. Now you are allowed to use the rest of the rows and you can integrate Saturday and Sunday as well. Plan your regeneration (use blue, please):

- Physical (i.e., course at a gym).
- Spiritual (i.e., schedule a walk alone, just for yourself, attend service according to your religion).
- Mental (i.e., book tickets for Fortuna Düsseldorf, plan to read, attend a concert).
- Social/emotional (plan and reserve time for your friends, partner).

For the remainder, use yellow: this is your spare and reserve time.

How does your week look like? Lots of blue? Lots of green? As a reference, check **Figs. 6.1** and **6.2**. Hopefully you were able to realize that despite your severe time restrictions (red and gray) you still have time resources that can be planned at your discretion. It is important to sit down and plan. Of course, the living reality will be quite different. But as long as you do not plan, you will not even realize that you have potential space for QII work.

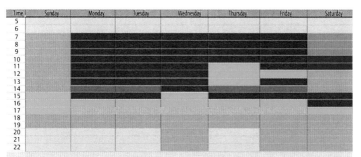

Fig. 6.1 A proposal for planning your week. Red: completely other-directed. Green: Quadrant II. Light gray: Quadrant I. Dark gray: Quadrant IV. Blue: regeneration. Yellow: spare and reserve.

Make it a habit to plan your week, every week. Reserve a slot for this as well. Put important QII items (i.e., project: discussion of paper. Action: read paper by Smith on brain plasticity) into the reserved spaces. Try to expand blue and green.

Be realistic. There will be a period of your life in which work demands are overwhelming and will squash your reserved time with yourself or your family. That might be very much okay, as long as you actively realize this and *plan* this. You might even decide to plan work on Saturday and Sunday. As long you feel comfortable with this, no problem. It might even be a relief to know that you can forward things at the end of a working day, when you are completely exhausted, to a relaxed hour in your office on Sunday afternoon. If you are controlling this, if you have decided that this is the way to do it and to plan it, you will even look forward to going to your office on Sunday, 4 PM. If you feel forced into spending an afternoon in the office, if you are not convinced, then you must absolutely not go.

Time	Sunday	Monday	Tuesday	Wednesday	Thursday	Friday	Saturday
5							
6							
7	Breakfast with family	Rounds	Rounds	Rounds	Rounds	Rounds	Breakfast with Family
8	Breakfast with family	OR	outpatient	Rounds	OR	OR	Breakfast with Family
9		OR	outpatient	ward work	OR	OR	
10		ward work	ward work	ward work	ward work	OR	Shopping
11		OR	outpatient		Review results of analysis (Project XY)	ward work	Shopping
12	Walk with partner and dog	OR	outpatient		Write report on PhD Thesis	Paper 1 Figures	Walk with partner and dog
13	Walk with partner and dog	OR	outpatient	Time off card	Call Head of Pathology: Cooperation	Time off card	Walk with partner and dog
14	Walk with partner and dog						Walk with partner and dog
15	weekly planning			Preparation Skills LAB			Cleaning house
16	sorting INBOX	Paper 1 Results	Paper 1 Results	Paper 1 Results	Write outline concept for funding		Work in garden
17	review projects	emails, calls	emails, calls	emails, calls	emails, calls	emails, calls	
18	GYM	Jogging	GYM	Jogging	GYM	Bicycle	Soccer
19	Dinner with family	Dinner with family	Dinner with family	Dinner with family	Dinner with family	Dinner with family	Soccer
20				Theatre		Friends	Soccer
21				Theatre		Friends	Friends
22				Theatre		Friends	Friends

Fig. 6.2 This is how a standard week could look like. Make it a habit to plan your week in detail. Focus on the green and do not forget how important blue is.

7 Acute Disaster Management: Three Major Points

The best way to cope with disaster is to prevent it in the first place.

Anonymous

When a disaster strikes, this "bon mot" is, however, as helpful for your actual situation as "I told you so."

What you need now are some efficient strategies to:

- Assess and contain the damage.
- Make the best out of the situation.
- Prevent it from happening again.

Let us assume that you are in an acute job-related crisis.

You have just realized that you did the skin incision on the wrong side.

How do you react? Wobbling knees? Vegetative reaction with profuse sweating? Verbal discharges (Fuck, Fuck, Fuck, "Typus Angloamericanus," Merda, Merda, Merda, "Typus Italianus," Mist, Mist, Mist, "Typus Germanicus," etc. You get the point)? It is understandable, but not helpful. Unfortunately, the next step is often to blame others: it is not my fault; the nurse put the drape on the wrong side, etc. This not only is unhelpful but also makes things worse, because you will lose the cooperation and respect of your coworkers and potentially start an argument.

7.1
Assess the Damage and Analyze the Situation

Now, what harm was done? What can you do to keep the damage as minor as possible?

In this situation, you will try to close the skin extra careful, and make extra sure that the planned procedure (on the correct side) will not have any further complications. You need to think about the potential legal consequences and how to approach the patient after surgery.

7.2
Make the Best Out of the Situation

Apart from making extra sure that the patient does not suffer from some further complications, you can actually draw some benefits from this situation. You can grow. By admitting that it was your responsibility, by honestly dealing with the patient and his relatives, and accepting a potential punishment, your professional personality can grow immensely.

7.3
Prevent It from Happening Again

This is the most important point. At a certain time, you need to do the postmortem (hopefully not literally). Find out what went wrong. Do not swear that this will not happen again; rather, install measures to prevent it. For the "wrong side" problem, the solution is obvious: stick to the time-out principle. Follow the checklist and check "side." Never touch "skin with knife" before running through your own mental checklist.

In the end, this disaster might have made you a better physician and a more mature personality.

I always tried to turn every disaster into an opportunity.

John D. Rockefeller

8 Anxiety Management: The "Power of Now" Approach

In a real dark night of the soul, it is always three o'clock in the morning, day after day.

F. Scott Fitzgerald

If you follow the principles described earlier, you should be in a mentally relaxed state of mind and at peace with yourself and the world. However, despite a perfect inbox and time matrix management, you will still be confronted with an accumulation of unsolved problems, uncontrolled situations, and uncomfortable "what if" thoughts. The accumulation of these little demons in your subconsciousness will eventually cost you: your peace of mind and (typically) your sleep.

In the hopefully rare situations, in which anxiety renders you ineffective and sleepless, a (pure) symptomatic "anxiolytic" approach is often very helpful. Your anxiety is most often related to an imaginary future situation. Allow yourself to accept that this future situation is just a mental phantom. It is not real. And it is absolutely not real in the present moment. Ask yourself what problem you have this second, in this moment.

Say, for example, you are worried about a presentation that you have to give. Typically, at 3 AM you wake up, your mind racing with nervous thoughts about a detail of slight 4. Your anxiety quickly spreads to other problems: you forgot the preparation of grand rounds in 2 days; you need to buy the vodka for the cocktail party on Saturday. You know that you will blow your next day if you do not get some sleep. Now consider what is wrong right now.

Nothing. You are in your bed, you can listen to the rain outside, you are absolutely safe, and nothing real is threatening you right now. It is all in your mind. None of the problems that you have can be solved right now. The best way to approach your problems is to understand this and go back to sleep. And, if you are really desperate and this does not work:

> *Even the darkest night will end and the sun will rise.*
> *(Victor Hugo)*

On the other hand, why do not you get up and start to solve your problem? It is up to you. You control the situation. Get some assurance from this thought as well. What you need to do is to get rid from unhealthy anxiety or even fear. Sometime ago, I came across Gaur Gopal Prabhu, an Indian lifestyle coach and a *brahmachari* (a man who practices *brahmacharya*, a type of living as per Hindu Vedic scriptures). In one of his lectures, he described in a very humorous way how to deal with problem-driven anxiety (**Fig. 8.1**).

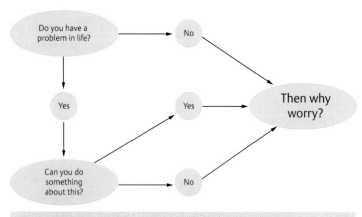

Fig. 8.1 Is this great wisdom? At least, it is funny.

It is very important that you realize that these approaches, however, are purely symptomatic. You do not solve your problems; you just cope with the situation for the sake of your peace of mind. The "Power of Now" approach is just a band aid for your soul. In the end, it is much more efficient to prevent threads by following the principles of proactivity, as described earlier. Try to cure, not to work on symptoms. Unfortunately, anxiety, and even fear, is often one of the major driving factors of our motivation—as long as it does not make you sick, you might take advantage of "healthy" anxiety and use it to boost your motivation. However, you walk a fine line there.

9 Networking

> *No man is an island, entire of itself; every man is a piece of the continent, a part of the main. If a clod be washed away by the sea, Europe is the less, as well as if a promontory were, as well as if a manor of thy friend's or of thine own were. Any man's death diminishes me because I am involved in mankind; and therefore never send to know for whom the bell tolls; it tolls for thee.*
>
> John Donne, Meditation XVII

Though this quotation from John Donne seems a little pathetic and has been used to introduce books on battles and heroism, it fits into certain aspects of residency. You are "brothers in arms"; you are a community in which the individual performance is indeed influencing the whole. You are part of a network. So let me make the case for altruism and teamwork. Despite your clear-cut goals and your defined career tract, you will need the support of your coworkers. In other words: if you do not have a sound fundament of trust and cooperation with your colleagues, you will be severely impaired in all aspects of your professional life. Unfortunately, high impact units often raise an atmosphere of competition, which might even lead to rivalry. This is often very counterproductive.

Let us assume that you find yourself in a rather unstructured unit where among the residents a spirit of mistrust, envy, and rivalry prevails.

"This is not my duty. If you guys don't do it: I will not step in." "This is typical for Dr. A: leaving the stuff for the guy on call, instead of doing it himself." "Why do I have to clean up after my colleagues?" "Why can he go to the OR and I have to stay on the ward?" "Why do I have to be on call on Christmas? Let Dr. B spent Christmas in the hospital." "Dr C. is uncooperative and always bad tempered and I cannot work with her on the same ward."

These are typical quotations of persons who work in a dysfunctional unit. Imagine the wasted time and energy that is spent for these struggles. Imagine that you need to do some experiments and the only person who can cover you is Dr. C (who has overheard you saying that she is uncooperative). You will have an unnecessary problem, which will eventually block you from going to the laboratory. No experiment, you will not publish the paper in time, you will therefore disqualify for the PhD program. You get the point.

It is therefore very advisable to invest time into building a functional team. Though this is a central task for the leadership of your unit, it is often neglected. As this is of genuine interest for you, consider to take the initiative.

What can you do?

- Define the problems:
  - Try to get an idea what is wrong by your own observation and by interviewing your colleagues. Make sure to be objective, most of all regarding your own position. Define the problems and draft some solutions.
- Raise the awareness for this problem:
  - Discuss with your colleagues in an individual approach the importance and impact of this unsatisfying situation.
- Find solutions:
  - Schedule a meeting with all persons involved. Define the major problems. Suggest performing a brainstorming

process regarding these topics. Summarize the discussion, and add your own observation.

- Offer your premeditated solutions.
- Run for your life.

Apart from actually having the chance to improve the situation in your department, you will train your leadership skills by this approach. It might make sense to have these meetings on a regular basis, maybe every month. You will hopefully observe a tendency toward increased socializing, comradeship, and even friendship.

It is worth noting that most of the highly professional teams in the commercial world take this team building and team fostering very seriously and spent substantial parts of their budget for team-building events. Companies expect higher productivity, better communication, and more creativity from these. It is pretty symptomatic for our (medical) professional culture that you rarely see groups of physicians on ropes and high wires, learning to safeguard each other.

10 The Mentor

As you start your residency, almost everybody will be more experienced than you. If the network in your department is functional, you will receive support from everybody until you have learned to swim. In this period, you will certainly realize that some of your colleagues (most likely the more senior ones) have a very impressive professional knowledge, are very influential, and are potentially representing exactly the position that you want to reach (according to your goals, see chapter "Goals"). This person knows everything about *how to get there*, can *help you to get there*, and can tell *how it is there*. It would be almost tragic for you and your career if you would not take advantage of this treasure. There are many very unprofessional ways to approach this pot of gold. Don't! The professional way is to ask for a mentorship. The idea of a mentorship is that a wise and trusted counselor or teacher supervises your career by counseling and support. In only very few (medical) departments, this is already implemented in the training program; it is therefore very likely that you need to take the initiative. How to approach this problem:

First of all, make sure that this person is in fact representing the goals that you are aiming at.

If you have identified the "chosen one," you need to approach the lucky person. It is now important that the mentor becomes interested in serving as a mentor. To this end, it is important that you:

- Know what you need and want from the mentorship.
- Have clearly defined goals.

- Identify problems you believe might be obstacles to you in reaching your goals.
- Give thought to and be able to articulate how you think a mentor could assist you.
- Think about how you might reach your goals with or without a mentor.
- Be purposeful and pleasant, and have challenging goals.

Treat your mentor relationship with care; do not abuse it by asking for inappropriate favors or support, and do not take your mentor for granted.

Mentors are volunteers; they do not get paid for their efforts. They do, however, want to receive some satisfaction from the mentoring. Somewhat similar to parents, a good mentor will hope to implement an important, long-lasting, positive impact on your life, an influence that helps you to move forward.

The only way that mentors can know how they are doing is if mentees tell them. What you have to offer your mentor is a feedback: your appreciation and an explanation of the impact the support of your mentor has had on your current and future success in life.

11 The Need for Reevaluation

11.1
Zooming In and Zooming Out

Your life is a very dynamic process. It is therefore very important that you repeat Exercises 1 to 8 on a regular basis. Schedule these repetitions as QII activities. By changing the perspective from *macro* to *micro*, you will make sure that you are still on the road to reach point B.

By this proactive approach, you will identify impending disasters.

Let us assume that you have the feeling that your job is not going so well. You are starting your third year as a resident and in your department a reevaluation is scheduled at the end of the third year. This evaluation will be crucial for the decision to offer you the next 3 years' contract. Elevate yourself into the macro position and review your travel from the first day to your actual position. Have you reached all the scheduled goals? What is missing?

- You might come up with a list of goals that you did not reach. Now follows a very important step. Answer these questions:

  a. Are these goals that you still need or want to reach?
     In fact, maybe the goal to reach a PhD degree is not important anymore. Maybe the performance of your first solo brain tumor operation is not important anymore, because you have decided to focus on spinal surgery. If your failure to achieve certain surgical skills at the target time point is not bothering you, maybe you

are not so eager to become a surgeon after all. So why bother with setting new surgical goal?

b. Are these crucial or minor goals? Assess the potential consequences of your failures.

c. Was it your fault or the fault of the system? Very important. And in answering this question, it is very important to be as honest and objective as possible. Since you might be hurt and emotional, you need an objective evaluation of the problem. It is very much possible that you are locked in the "if you do not like me, I do not like you" trap. Try to have your role and your perception of the system evaluated by a "third party." This could be your mentor or a colleague. This person might be hard to find, since she/he needs to be both objective and competent regarding your problem.

d. What were the reasons for your failure? Obviously, a very important question. As is the case with many postmortem examinations, the answer can be quite painful. They will, however, give you a unique opportunity to grow and to become a better person.

e. Can it be changed? Depending on your answer to d:
Or you need to change yourself: that is, work harder/ become more efficient, etc.
Or you have to change the system. Let us be realistic: you can criticize the system, but it is unlikely that you can change your training program. This might mean that you need to find another position in another hospital.

- You have fulfilled your plan but feel uneasy about your situation: up to the macro position and evaluate your goals. Are you running out of passion? Do you think a training program in a different hospital would promote your abilities more efficiently?

- You are fine: fine. As long as your boss thinks so as well. If criticism comes as a surprise, go back to section 1 and analyze your situation. You might need to say goodbye to as yet "essential" goals. These are potentially very painful processes. But they will keep your life as a whole on a track.

If you have fulfilled your plan, why are you feeling uneasy? Again, the macro perspective can clarify if you are still on track to the right goals. It is not uncommon that once you have reached your goals, you find out that you were mistaken in choosing these. Unfortunately, many of us stay on the wrong track because we are too inert to change.

12 The Art to Learn from Errors

On your way to learn and master one of the most complicated and demanding jobs, you will commit errors. Some of them will be so grave that you need disaster management and some so subtle that you will not realize these until someone else confronts you with your errors. On the other hand, you will do great—most of the tasks you accomplish will be a success and (especially as a physician) *you* personally will make the difference in other persons' lives. In one or another way, you will receive feedback for your actions. Your actions will be analyzed and evaluated. You are subject to two evaluation systems that are of utmost importance for your learning success: your medical environment (teacher, colleagues, patients, books, lectures, and so on) and yourself. During the learning process, you will commit errors. This is in the nature of things, inevitably and part of your educational process. Therefore, making errors is normal and not a catastrophe—as long as you learn from the errors and thus prevent them from happening again. To this end, several things need to happen.

First, you need to commit an error. Fine, thank you.

Ideally:

- Your environment or yourself or both systems will detect the error.
- The error will be communicated.
- The error will be analyzed.
- Prevent it from happening again.

Thus, the learning effect is maximized (**Fig. 12.1**). Unfortunately, this is rarely the case.

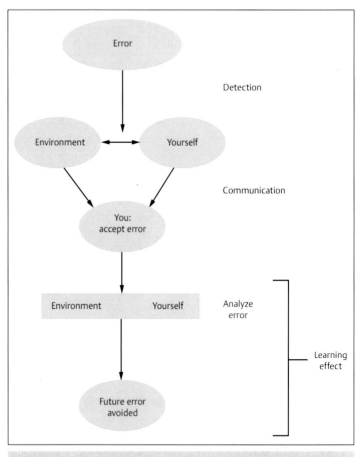

Fig. 12.1 The error cascade: detection–communication–learning effect: future error avoided.

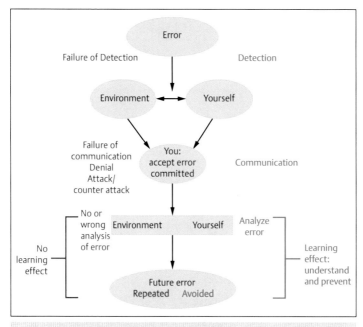

Fig. 12.2 What can go wrong if something went wrong.

Many things can go wrong (**Fig. 12. 2**):

1. Error will not be detected

A system that accepts "learning curves" must have implemented several checkpoints (checklists) that detect errors. You (yourself) and the environment are on the lookout for errors. An unintended incomplete resection of a tumor will be detected by postoperative imaging. This error is easy to detect. Inadequate soft skills, on the other hand, are much harder to uncover and can often not be detected by oneself.

2.   Failure of communication

The detected error must be communicated between both systems: this is obvious in cases in which one system is not aware of the error. For example:

- You are scheduled to perform an intervention that you are not yet able to perform. You need to report this error *to the environment*.
- You have terrible bedside manners. You find yourself adequate; the system sees you as an arrogant, coldhearted, nonempathic, and impolite rectal orifice (asshole). The environment needs to report this *to you*.

The crucial point is that in the end the information reaches you and that you accept the fact: error committed. Interestingly, you might be aware of your error, but deny it to yourself. Admitting to have committed an error is painful. Of course, we try to avoid getting hurt. Denial, thus pushing the problem away from our consciousness, below the surface of our mind, is a very common but nevertheless (very) big problem. It might give you some relief for the moment, but it is only postponing, not solving, the problem.

When we are confronted with our errors, we often feel that we are under attack, so we counterattack. This is a crucial point. It is quite understandable that upon criticism defense mechanisms kick in: "It was not me"; It is not my fault"; "I did not know that"; "I was too tired"; "there is no problem," "you are only saying this because you do not like me." Sounds familiar?

Attack: "Your work on the ward is sloppy, you have again forgotten to change the dressing in Room 34." Counterattack: "And you have forgotten to change the dressing in Room 35, you are sitting in glass house here." Counter-counter attack: "I cannot work with you, you are a lazy idiot and that's what everybody is thinking about you."

Let us assume that both dressings not made were the responsibility of attacker and counterattacker, respectively, and that the discussion went on for hours ending in shouting and calling of animal names. In conclusion: a tremendous loss of working time, ruined relationship, and no solution for the fact that on this particular ward patients with dressing have a problem. Most importantly, both idiots were far away from accepting that an error was committed.

As long as you are not able to communicate the error openly and honestly with yourself and your environment, you are not a mature personality, and as long as you have not accepted that you have committed an error, you will not be able to proceed and thus grow and learn.

3.   No/wrong analysis of error

A technical analysis of an error is often implemented in medical procedures, that is, the literally postmortem analysis or morbidity and mortality conferences. For the majorities of the (minor) errors committed during your residency, no standard operating procedure is established. Let us assume that the placement of a catheter in a body cavity (you choose the cavity, depending on your specialization) can in principle be done by a free-hand approach referring to anatomical landmarks. It is, however, more precise and safer to use ultrasound. You place the catheter and the position is suboptimal (completely wrong). The error is *detected* and *communicated*, and you have *accepted* that the catheter is in the wrong cavity (again, you choose the cavity, depending on your specialization). Obviously, you need to repeat the procedure and now you need to know exactly what went wrong. Otherwise, the error will be repeated.

So you sit down, analyze the procedure, and think about strategies to avoid the error:

Error: You did not use the ultrasound. Would the use of ultrasound have avoided the problem? Yes. Why did you not use it? You are not trained on the machine.

Solution: Get training.

Problem: You need to repeat the procedure today. Training needs time.

Solution: Ask a more experienced colleague to assist you.

Problem: You are reluctant to admit that you do not have the training.

Solution: Obvious. You need to be honest with yourself and learn to accept your situation. If you are building your education on compromises, the fundament will eventually crumble. At this point, you have the opportunity of tremendous personal growth. By openly admitting that you are not trained, you show courage and demonstrate to yourself and others that you are primarily interested in the cause and not in your selfishness. By the way, while discussing your problem with your superior you might find another error in the system.

Problem: There is no training program for ultrasound.

Solution: Establish a mandatory training program.

Epilogue

Nothing in this book is new. I am a brain (tumor) surgeon and have neither formal literary background nor formal psychological training. I quote from several books that I feel are a must-read and most of all I quote from my memories of more than 20 years of intense interactions in the field. I came across these books *not* by recommendation of my clinical teachers. And this is symptomatic for the situation of medical education: career planning and caring for your quality of life are not implemented in virtually any training programs. Why not? We allow you to open skulls, but we do not care about your value system. We put you under pressure, which is very likely to destroy your social connections, and we are not motivated to offer assistance and counseling. Is it because we did not have the privilege of this in our own education? We would never treat our patients like this. We apply the principle of survival of the fittest on a population of fine young physicians and accept a very high dropout rate. This is inhuman and an irresponsible handling of (human) resources. This book tries to change this, by teaching fundamental principles of self-organization. Hopefully, this book will help you during your development from inexperienced, insecure, and afraid to competent, relaxed, and experienced.

During this process, you will become a teacher yourself, a mentor, and maybe even a role model. Please remember how you started, how important it was to define goals, and how important it was to learn organizational skills and teach this. If anything in this book is of value to you, transfer the knowledge: teach! Do not let your colleagues reinvent the wheel; it is too costly for our patients, our families, and our quality of life.

Recommended Readings

Books

- Getting Things Done: The Art of Stress-Free Productivity. David Allen
- The 7 Habits of Highly Effective People: Restoring the Character Ethic. Stephen Covey
- Man's Search for Meaning, Viktor Frankl. Beacon Press, 2006

Apps

- Jamie's 20 Minute Meals. Jamie Oliver
- Nigella: The Quick Collection. Nigella Lawson
- You Are Your Own Gym: The Bible of Bodyweight Exercises. Mark Lauren

Recommended Video

Then why worry
https://youtu.be/ngLEhVU1Ezk?list=RDTQOKJsEu7EM

Recommended Software

Omnifocus © 2007–2016 The Omni Group

Reference

- Puchalski C, Ferrell B, Virani R, et al. Improving the quality of spiritual care as a dimension of palliative care: the report of the Consensus Conference. J Palliat Med 2009 Oct;12(10):885–904